Thriving v

A Guide to Assert

Cynthia   Matej

Copyright

Catalog

Introduction to Functional Neurological disorder

Functional Neurological Disorder (FND), sometimes referred to as Conversion Disorder, is a medical condition in which patients experience neurological symptoms such as paralysis, tremors, or seizures that cannot be explained by structural or physiological abnormalities in the brain or nervous system. These symptoms are real and can be debilitating, yet no clear neurological cause is identifiable through standard medical tests. This creates significant challenges both for the patient, who is often stigmatized, and for the medical community, which must distinguish FND from other, more easily diagnosable conditions. Despite its complexity, the recognition and treatment of FND are gaining more attention, as it is increasingly understood as a disorder involving a combination of neurological, psychological, and social factors.

1. Understanding Functional Neurological Disorder

FND falls under the broader category of somatic symptom disorders, in which patients experience physical symptoms that cannot be fully explained by medical tests. The hallmark of FND is the presence of neurological symptoms that do not have an identifiable organic cause. The disorder affects the normal functioning of the nervous system, causing symptoms that resemble those of neurological diseases, such as epilepsy, multiple sclerosis, or stroke. However, when doctors perform neurological examinations and tests, they find no evidence of structural damage or abnormalities in the brain or nervous system.

FND is not a psychological disorder per se, but it does often involve elements of mental and emotional distress. Patients with FND experience real, disabling symptoms such as loss of motor control, vision problems, abnormal sensations, or seizures, but these symptoms arise due to dysfunction in the brain's processing of physical signals rather than structural damage to the brain.

The symptoms of FND can vary significantly from person to person and may fluctuate in severity over time. The disorder is commonly seen in young to middle-aged adults, and while it can occur in children, it is more frequently diagnosed in adults.

2. Symptoms of Functional Neurological Disorder

The symptoms of FND are often divided into motor, sensory, and seizure-like symptoms, but the disorder is far more complex and varied than these categories suggest. The symptoms can mimic those of other neurological conditions, but unlike those conditions, they do not have identifiable physical causes.

a) Motor Symptoms:

Motor symptoms in FND may include:

Paralysis or Weakness: One of the most common symptoms of FND is motor paralysis or weakness in one or more parts of the body. This can range from partial weakness in a limb to complete paralysis of the affected area.

Tremors: Involuntary shaking or trembling of the limbs or other parts of the body is a common symptom, and it can be mistaken for essential tremor or Parkinson's disease.

Abnormal Gait: Patients may experience an unsteady gait, difficulty walking, or even an inability to walk due to weakness or lack of coordination.

Dystonia: This refers to abnormal, involuntary muscle contractions that lead to twisting or repetitive movements.

b) Sensory Symptoms:

Sensory symptoms in FND may include:

Numbness or Tingling: Patients may experience unusual sensations, such as tingling or numbness in different parts of the body.

Visual Disturbances: Vision may be impaired, including partial or complete loss of vision in one or both eyes. Double vision, blurred vision, and sensitivity to light are also common.

Pain: Some individuals with FND may experience chronic pain in various parts of their bodies, without an identifiable physical injury or condition.

c) Seizure-like Symptoms:

Seizure-like events, often called non-epileptic seizures or psychogenic seizures, can also be a significant symptom of FND. These seizures are similar in appearance to those seen in epilepsy but do not have the electrical brain activity associated with true epileptic seizures. They can cause jerking movements, loss of consciousness, and a variety of other symptoms that resemble epileptic seizures but are not caused by abnormal brain waves.

3. Causes and Mechanisms of FND

The exact causes of FND are not fully understood, but it is believed to result from a complex interaction of biological, psychological, and social factors. Researchers hypothesize that dysfunction in the brain's neural circuits leads to impaired communication between the brain and the body, resulting in physical symptoms that cannot be explained by traditional neurological or medical diagnoses.

a) Neurological Factors:

At the neurological level, abnormalities in brain function have been observed in patients with FND. Brain imaging studies using techniques such as functional magnetic resonance imaging (fMRI) and positron emission tomography (PET) have revealed that there may be altered patterns of brain activity in individuals with FND, particularly in areas responsible for motor control, emotion regulation, and sensory processing. However, these findings are often subtle and not present in every case, making it difficult to pinpoint a specific cause.

b) Psychological Factors:

While FND is not classified as a mental health disorder, psychological factors, particularly stress, trauma, and emotional distress, are strongly linked to the development and exacerbation of FND symptoms. Research has shown that patients with FND are more likely to have a history of psychological trauma, such as physical or sexual abuse, significant life stressors, or other forms of emotional distress. These psychological factors may lead to alterations in brain function, contributing to the development of physical symptoms.

c) Social and Environmental Factors:

Social and environmental factors can also play a role in the development of FND. For example, individuals who have experienced a lack of social support, difficulty coping with stress, or a history of chronic illness may be more vulnerable to developing FND. In some cases, patients may have a tendency to focus on physical symptoms as a way of coping with emotional or psychological stressors.

4. Diagnosis of FND

Diagnosing FND can be challenging due to the absence of clear biological markers and the overlap in symptoms with other neurological disorders. Doctors rely on careful patient history, neurological examination, and diagnostic tests to rule out other conditions before making a diagnosis of FND.

a) Exclusion of Other Conditions:

FND is a diagnosis of exclusion, meaning that it is made when other potential causes for the symptoms have been ruled out. This may involve a series of tests, including imaging studies (such as MRI or CT scans), blood tests, and electroencephalograms (EEG) to rule out conditions such as brain tumors, multiple sclerosis, epilepsy, or stroke.

b) Clinical Evaluation:

A thorough clinical evaluation is essential for diagnosing FND. This includes assessing the patient's medical history, understanding the onset and progression of symptoms, and conducting a physical and neurological exam. In some cases, specialized tests such as the Hoover's sign (a test for leg weakness) or the Babinski sign may be used to help differentiate between functional and organic neurological conditions.

c) Psychological Assessment:

Because psychological factors often play a role in FND, a psychological assessment may be part of the diagnostic process. This may involve interviews or questionnaires to assess the patient's mental health, stress levels, history of trauma, or other emotional concerns.

5. Treatment of FND

Treatment for FND is multifaceted and typically involves a combination of approaches, including physical therapy, psychological therapy, and medical management. Given that FND has both neurological and psychological components, treatment aims to address both aspects of the disorder.

a) Physical Therapy:

Physical therapy is often a crucial component of treatment for patients with FND. Occupational therapists and physiotherapists work with patients to improve motor function, mobility, and coordination. Techniques such as graded exposure, which involves gradually increasing physical activity levels, can help individuals regain control over their bodies and reduce functional impairment.

b) Cognitive Behavioral Therapy (CBT):

Psychological treatments, particularly Cognitive Behavioral Therapy (CBT), have shown promise in managing FND. CBT aims to help patients identify and modify unhelpful thought patterns and behaviors that may be exacerbating their symptoms. For instance, patients may learn how to reframe negative thoughts about their condition and develop coping strategies to reduce stress and emotional distress.

c) Multidisciplinary Approach:

A multidisciplinary approach, which involves collaboration between neurologists, psychologists, physical therapists, and other healthcare professionals, is often the most effective way to treat FND. This approach ensures that all aspects of the disorder, from neurological symptoms to psychological and social factors, are addressed.

d) Medication:

In some cases, medications may be used to manage symptoms associated with FND, particularly if the patient has underlying mental health conditions such as anxiety or depression. However, medications are not typically used to treat the primary symptoms of FND, and treatment is generally more focused on non-pharmacological approaches.

6. Prognosis and Outlook

The prognosis for individuals with FND can vary widely. Some patients experience significant improvement or even complete resolution of symptoms, particularly when treatment is initiated early and the condition is managed effectively. However, others may experience chronic or recurrent symptoms that can be debilitating. The course of the disorder is often unpredictable, with some individuals experiencing periods of symptom improvement followed by flare-ups.

Early intervention, a strong support system, and a comprehensive treatment plan that addresses both the neurological and psychological aspects of the disorder are essential to improving outcomes for individuals with FND.

7. Conclusion

Functional Neurological Disorder is a complex and often misunderstood condition that presents significant challenges for both patients and healthcare providers. While the symptoms of FND are real and can be profoundly disabling, they do not have an identifiable physical cause. The disorder is believed to arise from a combination of neurological, psychological, and social factors, and treatment requires a multidisciplinary approach that addresses all of these components.

With increased awareness and better understanding of FND, patients can receive more accurate diagnoses, appropriate treatments, and improved care. The road to recovery can be long, but with the right interventions, individuals with FND can regain control of their lives and manage their symptoms effectively. Continued research and advancements in neurobiology, psychology, and treatment strategies will further enhance the prognosis and quality of life for those affected by FND.

Your Brain and body and How these Link to symptoms

Functional Neurological Disorder (FND) is an illness that highlights the intricate connection between the brain and body. The symptoms of FND are a reflection of how the brain processes and interprets signals from the body, and how dysfunctions in that process can lead to physical manifestations. Unlike traditional neurological disorders, FND does not arise from visible, structural damage to the nervous system; rather, it occurs when the brain fails to correctly interpret or process information, leading to physical symptoms that seem neurologically based. Understanding this relationship between the brain and body in FND can offer insights into the symptoms people with the disorder experience.

1. The Brain-Body Connection: Basic Principles

The brain is the central command center of the body. It receives signals from all parts of the body, processes them, and then sends out appropriate responses that control physical functions such as movement, sensation, and cognition. The brain communicates with the body through a vast network of neurons, including the central nervous system (CNS), which consists of the brain and spinal cord, and the peripheral nervous system (PNS), which includes all other neural connections extending to muscles, organs, and tissues.

This sophisticated communication system allows the brain to monitor the body's condition and respond to internal and external stimuli. The way in which the brain processes sensory information — such as touch, pain, temperature, or proprioception (sense of body position) — and motor signals — such as voluntary movement and involuntary reflexes — is vital for normal function. When this system works well, the body moves, reacts, and functions in an integrated way. But when the communication between the brain and body breaks down, as it often does in FND, it can lead to the abnormal neurological symptoms observed in the disorder.

2. How FND Disrupts the Brain-Body Link

In FND, the brain's ability to process and coordinate body signals becomes disrupted. This does not mean that the brain is damaged in the traditional sense, such as in a stroke or multiple sclerosis. Instead, FND is associated with dysfunctional brain processing, where the brain fails to properly interpret or control physical responses. As a result, patients experience physical symptoms, such as paralysis, tremors, abnormal gait, or seizures, even though the neural pathways do not exhibit structural damage.

The brain, in essence, misinterprets normal signals or becomes "disconnected" from the sensory or motor information it receives. These "disruptions" can happen due to a variety of factors, including stress, trauma, emotional distress, or a history of neurological illness. The exact cause of these misinterpretations is not fully understood, but it's believed that the interaction between the brain's emotional processing centers (like the limbic system) and motor control centers (such as the motor cortex) plays a crucial role in the development of FND.

3. The Role of Stress and Emotions in FND

The emotional brain, specifically areas such as the amygdala and the hypothalamus, plays a crucial role in how the brain responds to stress and emotional triggers. These areas are involved in processing fear, anxiety, and other strong emotions. When someone experiences high levels of stress or emotional trauma, it can overload these brain centers and lead to disturbances in the neural pathways that manage physical movement and sensation.

For instance, stress can lead to an overactive fight-or-flight response, which in turn can cause a variety of physical manifestations, including muscle tension, heart palpitations, and even paralysis. In FND, this may result in motor symptoms such as weakness or tremors. This suggests that the physical symptoms of FND may be linked to the brain's abnormal processing of emotional states, turning psychological stress into physical dysfunction.

4. The Brain's Motor and Sensory Systems: Their Dysfunction in FND

The brain's motor system, located primarily in the motor cortex, is responsible for voluntary muscle control. In FND, patients may experience motor symptoms like weakness or paralysis, which often mimic conditions such as stroke or multiple sclerosis. However, in FND, imaging studies do not show structural damage to the brain or spinal cord.

Instead, the motor cortex's ability to send appropriate signals to the muscles may be impaired, resulting in symptoms such as functional paralysis or tremors. In some cases, the brain "forgets" how to properly use certain muscles, leading to what may appear as an involuntary limp or abnormal gait. This dysfunction can sometimes be triggered by psychological factors, with the brain incorrectly interpreting or "blocking" the motor function.

Similarly, the sensory systems, including those responsible for processing sensations like touch, pain, and temperature, may also be involved in FND. The somatosensory cortex, which is responsible for processing sensory input from the body, may become dysregulated. This could result in sensations such as numbness, tingling, or pain in the absence of any physical cause. A common phenomenon in FND is a sensory disturbance that affects specific body parts, such as the face or limbs, where the brain fails to interpret or perceive sensory input in a coherent way.

5. Seizure-like Symptoms: The Link Between Brain Misfiring and FND

Another striking symptom of FND is the occurrence of non-epileptic seizures (NES), which are seizures that resemble epileptic seizures but do not show the characteristic electrical discharges in the brain. These seizures are believed to occur when there is a miscommunication between the brain's seizure circuits and motor centers, causing abnormal motor movements or loss of consciousness without the typical electrical abnormality seen in epilepsy.

While traditional epilepsy is caused by abnormal electrical activity in the brain, NES in FND involves the brain processing dysfunction. The brain's circuitry, which normally keeps seizure activity in check, becomes disturbed. For instance, a person may have a seizure-like episode when under stress, anxiety, or emotional pressure, showing that stress and psychological factors can strongly influence the manifestation of these episodes.

This underscores the delicate relationship between the brain's emotional processing centers and motor control systems. The misfiring of neurons in these circuits leads to symptoms that mimic a neurological disorder but without a structural cause, as is seen in epilepsy.

6. The Psychological and Social Impact on the Brain-Body Link

Social and psychological factors, such as childhood trauma, chronic stress, life events, or negative experiences with medical professionals, can create a predisposition for FND. People who have experienced traumatic events or overwhelming stress may develop a hyperactive stress response system, leading to abnormal brain activity that manifests physically in the form of FND symptoms. This trauma can cause changes in the brain's wiring, especially in areas related to emotional regulation and bodily control, resulting in physical symptoms when emotional stress becomes too great.

Moreover, a history of mental health conditions like anxiety, depression, or post-traumatic stress disorder (PTSD) can make a person more vulnerable to FND. Emotional difficulties, such as fear of illness or heightened vigilance, can amplify the brain's misperception of sensory and motor signals, creating or worsening physical symptoms.

The brain's inability to separate physical and psychological symptoms often leads to a vicious cycle: patients experience physical symptoms (such as tremors or pain), which cause emotional distress, which in turn triggers more severe symptoms, perpetuating the disorder.

7. The Importance of Neuroplasticity in FND Recovery

The brain's remarkable ability to adapt and reorganize is known as neuroplasticity. While neuroplasticity is often associated with recovery from brain injuries or strokes, it is also a vital factor in conditions like FND. The brain can, in many cases, rewire its circuits and compensate for dysfunction, provided that the right treatment strategies are employed.

In the case of FND, treatments that focus on re-training the brain's motor and sensory circuits can be effective. Cognitive Behavioral Therapy (CBT), psychotherapy, and physical therapy aim to address the brain-body miscommunication by retraining the brain to correctly process physical and emotional signals. By targeting the brain's ability to adapt and "relearn" how to process and respond to sensory or motor information, these therapies help re-establish a healthy brain-body connection and reduce symptoms over time.

8. Conclusion

The brain and body are deeply interconnected, and the way the brain processes signals from the body is key to understanding the symptoms of Functional Neurological Disorder. FND arises when this connection is disrupted, often by a complex interaction of psychological, emotional, and physiological factors. The symptoms of FND are real and reflect an underlying dysfunction in brain activity rather than structural damage. Through multidisciplinary treatment approaches, including psychological therapy and physical rehabilitation, the brain's ability to process and respond to bodily signals can be restored, allowing individuals with FND to recover and regain normal function. Understanding this brain-body link is essential to supporting individuals with FND and improving their quality of life.

Five Areas Approach to improving Things

The Five Area Approach is a practical and structured method that can be applied to improving the lives of individuals with Functional Neurological Disorder (FND). This disorder, characterized by neurological symptoms without a clear structural cause, can be deeply impactful on a person's daily life. The Five Area Approach focuses on addressing key factors that influence FND and aims to improve overall well-being by targeting the Mental, Physical, Skills, Social, and Strategic aspects of a person's life. Here's how this approach can be tailored to individuals with FND to improve their symptoms and quality of life.

1. Mental Area (Mindset, Thoughts, and Emotional Health)

A positive mental or psychological framework is central to managing FND. Since FND can often be triggered or exacerbated by emotional stress, anxiety, and trauma, addressing the mental area can have profound effects on symptoms.

Focus Areas:

Cognitive Behavioral Therapy (CBT): This therapeutic approach is especially useful in FND treatment. It helps individuals recognize and challenge unhelpful thought patterns and beliefs that may contribute to their symptoms. CBT can be used to reduce anxiety, depression, and stress, all of which are common among FND patients.

Mindfulness and Stress Management: Techniques such as mindfulness meditation, deep breathing, and progressive muscle relaxation can help reduce stress levels. Stress is a known trigger for many FND symptoms, so learning to manage emotional responses can help mitigate their impact.

Resilience and Coping Strategies: Building resilience by focusing on problem-solving and developing effective coping strategies can help patients deal with the psychological and emotional challenges that accompany FND. These strategies can improve mental well-being and foster a positive outlook despite ongoing symptoms.

Outcome:

Improved emotional regulation and a shift in mindset can reduce the severity of FND symptoms and improve a person's ability to cope with the challenges of the disorder.

2. Physical Area (Body, Movement, and Sensory Processing)

The physical symptoms of FND—such as paralysis, tremors, weakness, or non-epileptic seizures—are often manifestations of the brain's miscommunication with the body. The physical area focuses on improving movement, mobility, and addressing any physical health concerns related to FND.

Focus Areas:

Physical Therapy (PT): Tailored physical therapy can help improve motor function, strength, coordination, and movement patterns. It can be particularly beneficial for individuals experiencing functional weakness, tremors, or gait disturbances. PT helps retrain the body to move correctly and build physical strength.

Occupational Therapy (OT): Occupational therapists help individuals with FND develop strategies to manage daily activities, such as dressing, cooking, or working. They can also help improve fine motor skills and cognitive motor skills.

Neuromuscular Retraining: Certain forms of therapy, such as sensory integration therapy, can address issues in sensory processing. By gradually and safely exposing individuals to specific stimuli, therapists can help retrain the brain's processing of sensory information, improving the accuracy of sensory responses.

Exercise Programs: Exercise can be helpful in improving overall physical health, boosting energy levels, and reducing symptoms related to stress and anxiety. A tailored exercise program can help individuals regain strength and confidence in their physical capabilities.

Outcome:

Improved physical functioning, enhanced motor skills, and better sensory processing can lead to a reduction in functional symptoms such as tremors, weakness, and seizures. Physical interventions can also foster greater independence in daily life.

3. Skills Area (Cognitive, Coping, and Functional Skills)

People with FND may experience cognitive challenges such as memory problems, difficulty concentrating, or processing information. Additionally, they may need to improve skills to manage their symptoms and daily activities effectively.

Focus Areas:

Cognitive Rehabilitation: Cognitive rehabilitation strategies, often used for conditions like brain injury or stroke, can be beneficial in FND. These therapies help individuals develop better cognitive function by retraining the brain to improve attention, memory, problem-solving, and executive functions.

Skills for Managing FND Symptoms: Developing specific skills for managing FND symptoms can empower individuals to regain control over their condition. This includes strategies for handling non-epileptic seizures, functional movement disorders, and other functional symptoms.

Self-management Programs: Teaching individuals coping strategies to manage their condition daily, including pacing, stress reduction techniques, and using adaptive tools, can improve overall quality of life. Self-management skills can help individuals handle fluctuations in symptoms more effectively.

Outcome:

By enhancing cognitive abilities, improving self-management skills, and equipping individuals with strategies to cope with FND symptoms, patients may experience greater functional independence and less interference from their symptoms in daily activities.

4. Social Area (Relationships, Support Networks, and Communication)

The social aspect of FND is often underestimated but is crucial to the individual's well-being. Social interactions and support networks play a significant role in a person's ability to manage their condition and live a fulfilling life. This area focuses on improving relationships, communication, and social support.

Focus Areas:

Support Networks: Building strong support networks is key for individuals with FND. This could involve family, friends, healthcare professionals, and support groups. Having people to rely on can provide emotional support, reduce isolation, and offer practical assistance when needed.

Education for Family and Friends: Educating loved ones about FND can help them better understand the condition, how to offer support, and how to respond to symptoms in a way that is helpful. This reduces misunderstandings and promotes a more supportive environment.

Community and Peer Support: Peer support groups for FND can offer a sense of camaraderie and understanding. Sharing experiences with others facing similar challenges can help reduce feelings of isolation and provide practical tips for managing symptoms.

Improved Communication: Encouraging open and honest communication with healthcare providers and support networks is essential. Effective communication helps ensure that individuals with FND feel heard and understood, leading to more personalized care and support.

Outcome:

Strengthening social connections, fostering supportive relationships, and increasing social understanding can improve emotional well-being and reduce the stigma associated with FND. A well-established support system can help individuals with FND navigate their condition more effectively.

5. Strategic Area (Planning, Goal-Setting, and Medical Management)

The strategic area focuses on establishing clear, actionable plans for managing FND and improving long-term health outcomes. This includes goal-setting, medical management, and interdisciplinary care.

Focus Areas:

Interdisciplinary Team Approach: Collaboration between neurologists, psychologists, physical therapists, occupational therapists, and other healthcare providers is key in managing FND. A comprehensive, integrated treatment plan that addresses both physical and psychological aspects of FND is often the most effective approach.

Personalized Treatment Plans: Tailored treatment plans that account for the unique symptoms and triggers of each individual with FND are essential. This includes adjusting therapies as needed and making modifications based on the individual's progress.

Setting Short-term and Long-term Goals: Establishing clear, realistic goals—both short-term and long-term—can help individuals with FND stay motivated and track their progress. These goals could range from improving mobility or reducing specific symptoms to managing stress more effectively.

Regular Monitoring and Adjustments: Ongoing assessment of symptoms and treatment outcomes helps ensure that the person with FND is receiving the most effective care. Adjusting strategies and interventions as needed can lead to sustained improvement.

Outcome:

A clear plan for medical care, rehabilitation, and personal goals, alongside an organized approach to managing symptoms, can promote better control over FND symptoms and lead to measurable progress over time.

Conclusion

The Five Area Approach to improving Functional Neurological Disorder (FND) provides a holistic, comprehensive framework for managing the disorder. By addressing the mental, physical, skills, social, and strategic aspects of the condition, individuals with FND can achieve a more balanced and effective recovery. The key to success lies in addressing the interplay between these areas, understanding that improvement in one domain often supports progress in others.

Implementing this approach requires a multi-faceted treatment plan that includes psychological therapies, physical rehabilitation, skill-building, social support, and clear medical strategies. With a tailored, integrated approach, individuals with FND can improve their quality of life, reduce symptom severity, and regain a sense of control over their daily lives.

Behaviours

In the context of Functional Neurological Disorder (FND), behaviors can refer to the various physical, emotional, and psychological responses individuals exhibit as a result of their condition. These behaviors may manifest as part of the disorder itself, due to how the brain processes and responds to sensory or motor input, or as a way to cope with the challenges associated with living with FND.

Types of Behaviors in FND

1. Physical Behaviors (Motor Symptoms)

One of the key features of FND is the presence of motor symptoms that mimic neurological conditions such as paralysis, tremors, and abnormal movements. These symptoms, however, are not the result of underlying neurological damage but rather a disruption in the brain's ability to process motor signals.

Examples of physical behaviors include:

Functional Weakness: This behavior may present as paralysis or weakness in certain body parts, despite no evidence of structural damage to the nerves or muscles. Individuals may exhibit difficulty in moving limbs or even walking.

Tremors: Uncontrollable shaking or trembling, often without an identifiable cause. These tremors may occur during specific activities or continuously.

Functional Seizures: Non-epileptic seizures are seizure-like episodes that do not involve the typical electrical discharges seen in epilepsy. These may include shaking, loss of consciousness, or convulsions.

Gait Abnormalities: People with FND may develop an abnormal walking pattern, such as dragging a leg or shuffling.

Dystonia: Abnormal muscle contractions or postures that may cause twisting movements, often affecting specific parts of the body.

2. Psychological and Emotional Behaviors The psychological aspect of FND plays a critical role in symptom development and maintenance. Mental health factors such as anxiety, depression, trauma, and stress often influence the onset or severity of FND symptoms. Additionally, patients might exhibit certain coping behaviors as they deal with their symptoms.

Examples of psychological and emotional behaviors include:

Anxiety and Fear Responses: Individuals with FND may have intense fears regarding their symptoms or condition, leading to avoidance behaviors. For example, they may avoid social situations or certain activities due to fear of triggering symptoms like seizures or tremors.

Catastrophizing: This is a form of negative thinking where an individual may assume the worst possible outcomes for their condition, leading to heightened anxiety and increased physical symptoms. This behavior can hinder recovery as it amplifies the focus on symptoms.

Hypervigilance: People with FND may become overly focused on their body and symptoms, constantly monitoring their physical state for any signs of worsening. This heightened awareness can lead to increased stress and a sense of helplessness.

Depressive Behaviors: Feelings of helplessness, sadness, or hopelessness can lead to withdrawal from activities or social interactions. People with FND may isolate themselves due to perceived limitations or fear of judgment from others.

3. Coping Behaviors Coping behaviors are the strategies individuals use to manage the emotional and physical challenges of FND. While some of these coping strategies can be adaptive, others may contribute to a cycle of distress and exacerbate symptoms.

Examples of coping behaviors include:

Avoidance: Avoiding activities that may trigger symptoms (like physical exertion or social engagements) may be a common behavior. While avoidance can provide temporary relief, it can lead to further physical deconditioning, social isolation, and psychological distress.

Overcompensation: Some individuals may engage in overcompensation by pushing themselves beyond their limits in an effort to "prove" they can still function, even when this results in increased symptom severity or exhaustion.

Reassurance-Seeking: Repeatedly seeking reassurance from medical professionals, family members, or friends about the symptoms or condition may be a common coping behavior. This can become a way of dealing with the uncertainty of FND, though it may prevent patients from learning how to self-manage or trust their own judgment.

4. Social Behaviors Social behaviors in individuals with FND may be influenced by the fear of judgment, lack of understanding from others, or the limitations imposed by their symptoms. These behaviors can impact relationships with family, friends, colleagues, and healthcare providers.

Examples of social behaviors include:

Withdrawal or Isolation: Individuals with FND may withdraw from social situations or relationships due to embarrassment or fear of not being believed or understood. Social isolation can contribute to emotional distress and worsen symptoms.

Stigma and Misunderstanding: Due to the nature of FND— where there is no clear physical pathology visible— individuals may experience disbelief or skepticism from others. This can lead to frustration or anger, and some individuals may react defensively or avoid discussing their condition with others.

Seeking External Validation: In some cases, individuals with FND may become dependent on external validation to confirm their experiences or struggles. This behavior could involve seeking constant attention or acknowledgment from others about the severity of symptoms.

5. Functional Maladaptive Behaviors In some cases, individuals with FND may engage in behaviors that inadvertently reinforce or maintain their symptoms. These maladaptive behaviors can become ingrained over time and make it more challenging for the person to recover.

Examples include:

Reinforcement of the Sick Role: Sometimes, patients may adopt a passive "sick role" behavior, which involves focusing excessively on the diagnosis and symptoms, potentially preventing them from taking active steps toward recovery. This can be inadvertently reinforced by caregivers or medical professionals who focus solely on symptom management.

Unconscious Behavior Patterns: Some individuals may subconsciously develop behaviors such as "playing down" their symptoms or avoiding certain movements in anticipation of pain or discomfort. These ingrained patterns can hinder the recovery process and make it difficult for the brain to reestablish normal motor or sensory function.

Understanding and Modifying Behaviors in FND

Treatment Approaches to Address Maladaptive Behaviors:

1. Psychotherapy: Psychological treatments, such as Cognitive Behavioral Therapy (CBT) and Acceptance and Commitment Therapy (ACT), can help individuals with FND identify and modify maladaptive behaviors, thoughts, and emotions. CBT helps individuals challenge irrational beliefs about their symptoms and teaches them healthier coping mechanisms, while ACT focuses on accepting the presence of symptoms and committing to meaningful actions despite them.

2. Behavioral Therapy: In addition to traditional psychotherapy, specific behavioral therapies can be used to modify problematic behaviors, particularly avoidance or overcompensation. Techniques like exposure therapy may be helpful for confronting fears around physical activity, social situations, or movement.

3. Physical and Occupational Therapy: Therapy can help retrain motor functions, encourage mobility, and break avoidance cycles. It can also address functional behaviors like maladaptive posture, gait, or movements that may have developed in response to FND symptoms.

4. Family Therapy and Support: Educating family members about FND and how to provide effective support can help mitigate social withdrawal and emotional distress. A supportive family environment can encourage positive social behaviors and help patients maintain social connections despite the challenges of the disorder.

5. Mindfulness and Stress Reduction: Mindfulness practices, such as mindfulness meditation, breathing exercises, and progressive muscle relaxation, can help individuals gain better control over their thoughts and emotions, reducing the stress that contributes to maladaptive behaviors.

Conclusion

Behaviors in Functional Neurological Disorder (FND) are multifaceted and can range from physical manifestations of the condition, like tremors and paralysis, to emotional and social reactions, such as anxiety or social withdrawal. These behaviors are often a result of the brain's misinterpretation of signals and the impact of psychological stressors, trauma, or anxiety. Recognizing and addressing these behaviors through integrated treatments—including psychotherapy, physical therapy, social support, and behavioral modifications—can significantly improve outcomes for individuals with FND. By targeting maladaptive behaviors and promoting healthier coping strategies, individuals with FND can experience better symptom management and an improved quality of life.

Noticing and changing Unhelpful thinking

Noticing and Changing Unhelpful Thinking is a key component of managing Functional Neurological Disorder (FND) and many other mental health conditions. In FND, individuals may experience distressing physical and psychological symptoms that can lead to patterns of unhelpful thinking. These thought patterns often exacerbate symptoms, increase stress, and impede recovery. The good news is that with appropriate techniques, it's possible to identify these unhelpful thoughts and replace them with healthier, more constructive ones. Below is a guide on how to notice and change unhelpful thinking.

What is Unhelpful Thinking?

Unhelpful thinking refers to negative, distorted, or irrational thought patterns that can affect how we perceive ourselves, our symptoms, and the world around us. These thoughts often lead to feelings of anxiety, depression, and hopelessness, which can worsen FND symptoms, create barriers to recovery, and reduce the quality of life.

Some examples of unhelpful thinking include:

Catastrophizing: Imagining the worst-case scenario, assuming that things will go wrong or get worse.

Overgeneralizing: Taking one instance or event and making broad conclusions that apply to everything.

Black-and-White Thinking: Viewing situations, symptoms, or experiences as all good or all bad, with no room for nuance or complexity.

Mind Reading: Believing that others are thinking negatively about you or judging you without any actual evidence.

Personalization: Blaming yourself for things that are not your fault or believing that everything revolves around you.

Emotional Reasoning: Believing that because you feel a certain way, it must be true (e.g., "I feel helpless, so I must be helpless").

Why is Noticing and Changing Unhelpful Thinking Important in FND?

Unhelpful thinking in FND can increase emotional distress and make physical symptoms worse. For example:

Catastrophizing about your symptoms (e.g., "I'll never get better") can increase feelings of hopelessness and anxiety, which may worsen physical symptoms like tremors or seizures.

Overgeneralizing by thinking that all medical professionals or treatments are ineffective ("No treatment has worked for me, so nothing ever will") can prevent you from seeking or persisting with helpful treatments.

Mind reading and assuming that others are not empathetic can lead to isolation and a lack of social support.

By noticing and changing unhelpful thinking patterns, individuals with FND can improve their emotional well-being, reduce stress, and break the cycle of negative thoughts that exacerbate their symptoms.

Step-by-Step Guide to Noticing and Changing Unhelpful Thinking

1. Become Aware of Your Thoughts (Noticing)

The first step to changing unhelpful thinking is becoming aware of your thought patterns. This requires paying attention to your internal dialogue, particularly when you're feeling stressed, anxious, or frustrated. Mindfulness techniques can be helpful here.

How to Become Aware of Your Thoughts:

Mindfulness Practice: Set aside time each day to practice mindfulness, which involves focusing on the present moment without judgment. Mindfulness allows you to observe your thoughts and emotions without being overwhelmed by them.

Thought Journaling: Keep a journal where you write down your thoughts, especially during moments of emotional distress. Writing can help you notice recurring patterns of negative thinking.

Check-in with Yourself: Periodically ask yourself, "What am I thinking right now?" during moments of discomfort or symptom flare-ups. Pay attention to any automatic thoughts that arise, such as worrying about your symptoms or assuming the worst about your recovery.

Example: If you experience a tremor or other physical symptom of FND, you might notice a thought like, "This is going to get worse, and I'll never be able to function normally again." This is a form of catastrophizing, which is an unhelpful thought pattern.

2. Challenge the Thought (Examining Evidence)

Once you've identified an unhelpful thought, the next step is to challenge it. This involves examining the evidence for and against that thought, and considering whether there might be another, more balanced way of thinking about the situation.

How to Challenge Unhelpful Thoughts:

Ask, "Is this thought based on facts or assumptions?" Try to separate facts from assumptions. For example, "There's no evidence to suggest that my symptoms will keep getting worse in the long term."

Look for evidence to the contrary: Ask yourself, "Has there been a time when my symptoms improved? Have I had good days? What things have helped me in the past?" Remembering positive instances or progress, no matter how small, can provide a more balanced perspective.

Consider alternative explanations: "Could there be other reasons for my symptoms besides what I'm assuming? Could it be that I need more time to recover?"

Example: If you're thinking, "I'll never get better," ask yourself: "Have there been times when I felt better? Have doctors or therapists told me that progress is possible?" This helps you to challenge the idea that improvement is impossible.

3. Reframe the Thought (Creating a Balanced Perspective)

After challenging the negative or unhelpful thought, the next step is to reframe it into something more balanced or realistic. This involves replacing the irrational, negative thought with a more constructive, helpful one.

How to Reframe Unhelpful Thoughts:

Create a balanced alternative thought: Instead of thinking, "I'll never get better," reframe the thought as, "Recovery is a process, and I've made progress. Some days are better than others, but there's always hope."

Focus on what you can control: Change your focus from things that are outside your control to things that are within your control. For example, instead of thinking, "I can't control my symptoms," think, "I can control how I respond to my symptoms, and I can use coping strategies to manage my anxiety."

Use affirmations or positive self-talk: Create positive statements that are supportive and realistic. For example, "I may be struggling right now, but I am taking steps to improve my health and well-being."

Example: If your thought is "My symptoms will never go away," try reframing it to: "My symptoms may improve with time and treatment. I have learned how to manage them better and am continuing to work on my health with the help of my doctors."

4. Test and Evaluate the New Thought (Behavioral Experiment)

Once you've reframed your unhelpful thought, the next step is to test the new, more balanced perspective. This involves taking actions based on the new thought and seeing how it affects your behavior and feelings.

How to Test the New Thought:

Act as if the new thought is true: For example, if your new thought is "Recovery is possible and I am making progress," you can try engaging in an activity that you might usually avoid, such as going for a walk or trying a new coping strategy.

Evaluate the outcome: After testing the new thought, reflect on how you felt. Did you feel better after taking action based on the new thought? Did the new behavior help to reduce your symptoms or improve your mood?

Example: If you are fearful of going out in public because of potential seizures or other symptoms, you could test the new thought ("I can manage my symptoms and take breaks if needed") by gradually reintroducing social activities in a controlled way. Reflect afterward to see how your anxiety and symptoms were impacted by the experience.

5. Reinforce Positive Thinking and Make it a Habit

The final step is to make noticing and changing unhelpful thinking a regular part of your routine. Over time, these new patterns of thinking can become automatic, helping you to manage FND more effectively.

How to Reinforce New Thought Patterns:

Practice regularly: Like any skill, changing thinking patterns takes time and consistent practice. Make a habit of checking in with your thoughts and challenging unhelpful thinking every day.

Celebrate small wins: Acknowledge when you notice a shift in your thinking or when a new, balanced perspective leads to improved well-being. Small steps lead to lasting change.

Example: If you successfully challenge a negative thought like "I'm never going to get better" and replace it with "I am making progress every day," continue practicing this new thought by reaffirming it regularly. Keep a journal of your successes to reinforce the habit.

Conclusion

Noticing and changing unhelpful thinking is a powerful tool for managing Functional Neurological Disorder (FND). By becoming aware of negative thought patterns, challenging them, reframing them into more realistic perspectives, and testing those perspectives through behavior, individuals can break the cycle of distress that often accompanies FND symptoms.

Incorporating these techniques into daily life, along with support from healthcare providers, can help individuals feel more empowered in their recovery and improve both their mental and physical well-being. Over time, this can lead to a greater sense of control, reduced anxiety, and a more positive outlook on the future.

Overcoming Reduced activity and avoidance

Reduced activity and avoidance are common behavioral responses in individuals with Functional Neurological Disorder (FND), but they can exacerbate symptoms and hinder recovery. These behaviors are often driven by the fear of triggering symptoms, anxiety, or frustration about physical limitations. While they may offer short-term relief, in the long run, they can increase disability, worsen emotional distress, and perpetuate a cycle of avoidance and inactivity. Overcoming reduced activity and avoidance is crucial for improving both physical and psychological well-being in FND.

In this section, we'll explore how to recognize avoidance and inactivity patterns, understand their impact, and introduce strategies to overcome these behaviors to promote recovery and enhance quality of life.

Understanding Reduced Activity and Avoidance

Reduced Activity

Reduced activity refers to a decrease in physical, social, or emotional engagement due to the symptoms of FND. This reduction can occur across various domains:

Physical Activity: Individuals may avoid exercise or movement because of fears that it might trigger physical symptoms (such as tremors, seizures, or pain).

Social Activity: People may withdraw from social engagements due to embarrassment, anxiety, or the uncertainty of how others will react to their symptoms.

Work or Educational Activities: Individuals may avoid returning to work or school due to a lack of confidence in their ability to perform tasks or concerns about their symptoms being noticed or misunderstood.

Avoidance

Avoidance behavior involves deliberately steering clear of situations, environments, or activities that might provoke discomfort or anxiety. In the context of FND, this could include:

Avoiding physical exertion because it may lead to symptom flare-ups.

Avoiding social situations to prevent embarrassment or judgment.

Avoiding certain environments (e.g., busy places) to reduce sensory overload or stress.

Avoiding confrontation with one's symptoms, which may include refusing to engage in activities that challenge the limits imposed by the disorder.

While avoidance may seem like a protective mechanism, it can reinforce feelings of helplessness, reinforce disability, and limit opportunities for recovery and improvement.

Why Overcoming Avoidance and Reduced Activity Is Important

1. Physical Deconditioning: When individuals with FND reduce their physical activity, it can lead to physical deconditioning. This makes muscles weaker, reduces coordination, and diminishes endurance, which can increase the severity of symptoms and perpetuate the cycle of inactivity.

2. Psychological Impact: Avoidance and reduced activity can worsen feelings of anxiety, depression, and isolation. Social withdrawal due to FND symptoms can lead to loneliness, which may further exacerbate the psychological impact of the disorder. Avoidance of challenges can reinforce the belief that one is incapable, which can lower self-esteem and self-efficacy.

3. Increased Disability: Avoidance of activities that might trigger symptoms often results in further functional

decline. When individuals avoid challenging themselves, they miss opportunities to rebuild confidence, regain lost functions, and improve their quality of life.

4. Loss of Control: Over time, avoidance and reduced activity can lead to a feeling of losing control over one's life and daily activities. This helplessness can increase anxiety and perpetuate the belief that FND symptoms define the individual's capabilities.

Strategies to Overcome Reduced Activity and Avoidance

1. Gradual Exposure and Activity Reintroduction

One of the most effective ways to overcome avoidance behaviors is through gradual exposure. This involves slowly and systematically reintroducing activities or situations that have been avoided due to fear or anxiety. Gradual exposure helps to reduce fear and build confidence.

How to Use Gradual Exposure:

Start Small: Begin with tasks that are slightly challenging but not overwhelming. For example, if you've been avoiding exercise due to fear of triggering symptoms, you might start with a short walk or light stretching. Gradually increase the duration and intensity as you build confidence.

Set Realistic Goals: Break down larger activities or tasks into manageable steps. For example, if returning to work or school seems overwhelming, start by attending for half a day or working from home initially.

Monitor Progress: Keep track of your progress over time, and celebrate small victories. Gradual exposure helps desensitize the fear around certain activities, making them feel less threatening.

Example: If you're afraid of going to a busy place due to the fear of overwhelming symptoms (such as seizures), start by visiting less crowded areas, gradually increasing exposure to busier environments. You can also take breaks when needed and use relaxation techniques to manage anxiety.

2. Build a Routine

A structured routine provides a sense of control and stability, which can combat the unpredictability that often accompanies FND. A well-planned routine that incorporates both rest and activity can help reduce feelings of overwhelm and ensure that you're making consistent progress.

How to Build a Routine:

Include Rest Periods: Make sure that your routine is not too rigid or exhausting. Incorporate periods of rest to avoid physical and mental burnout, especially when returning to activity after a period of reduced engagement.

Balance Activities: Plan for a balance between physical, social, and cognitive activities. For example, after attending a social event, you might rest or engage in a low-energy activity to help prevent exhaustion.

Flexibility: Be flexible in your routine, allowing for changes if symptoms worsen or if you're feeling unwell. The goal is to maintain some level of engagement without overwhelming yourself.

Example: Start your day with a routine that includes light stretching, a healthy breakfast, and a small social activity (like calling a friend). As you feel stronger, you can increase the complexity of the activities.

3. Cognitive Behavioral Therapy (CBT)

CBT is highly effective for overcoming unhelpful thought patterns that contribute to avoidance and reduced activity. It helps individuals challenge negative beliefs and develop healthier, more realistic thinking about their symptoms and abilities.

How CBT Can Help:

Identifying Cognitive Distortions: CBT helps individuals identify negative or irrational thoughts related to activity (e.g., "If I try to exercise, I'll make my symptoms worse"). These thoughts are then replaced with more balanced, helpful beliefs (e.g., "Exercise can help improve my strength and reduce my symptoms in the long term").

Addressing Anxiety: CBT techniques such as exposure therapy can help reduce anxiety by gradually confronting feared situations (such as physical exertion or social engagement).

Building Self-Efficacy: CBT helps improve confidence in one's ability to cope with symptoms and handle life's challenges, which directly counteracts avoidance and inactivity.

Example: If you avoid exercise because of fear that it will worsen symptoms, CBT might help you reframe that belief to something like, "While exercise may be challenging, it can improve my physical function over time and I can modify my routine to suit my abilities."

4. Activity Pacing and Energy Management

One reason for avoidance and reduced activity in FND is the fear of fatigue or symptom exacerbation. Learning to pace activities and manage energy can help prevent this cycle of avoidance.

How to Pace Activities:

Break Tasks into Smaller Steps: Divide larger activities into smaller, more manageable tasks, and take breaks in between.

Rest Strategically: Ensure that you schedule breaks throughout the day to rest and prevent physical or mental exhaustion.

Monitor Symptoms: Pay attention to the signs of fatigue or symptom escalation, and take rest breaks as needed.

Example: If walking for 10 minutes causes fatigue or worsens symptoms, start with 5-minute walks and gradually increase the duration as your body adapts. Balance physical activity with periods of rest, and ensure you don't push yourself beyond your limits.

5. Social Support

Having support from family, friends, or a therapeutic community is essential when overcoming reduced activity and avoidance. Social support provides encouragement, reduces isolation, and creates opportunities for engagement in social or recreational activities.

How to Engage Social Support:

Share Your Challenges: Communicate openly with family or friends about your goals and limitations. Their support can help you feel more confident in returning to activities.

Join a Support Group: Consider joining a group for individuals with FND or chronic health conditions. This provides a safe space to share experiences and gain insights from others who understand your challenges.

Engage in Activities with Others: Involve friends or family in activities that feel manageable, like short walks, attending support groups, or doing activities you enjoy together. Socializing with others can also help reduce anxiety and isolation.

Example: Invite a friend or family member to accompany you for a walk or to attend a social event. Their presence provides reassurance and reduces the anxiety that might otherwise lead to avoidance.

Conclusion

Overcoming reduced activity and avoidance is crucial for recovery from Functional Neurological Disorder (FND). By understanding the impact of these behaviors and implementing strategies such as gradual exposure, CBT, routine building, activity pacing, and social support, individuals with FND can begin to break the cycle of inactivity and avoidance. These strategies empower individuals to reclaim control over their lives, reduce symptoms, and ultimately enhance their quality of life.

Consistency, patience, and a willingness to gradually challenge yourself are key to overcoming these barriers. With time, individuals with FND can rebuild confidence in their abilities, improve physical and emotional well-being, and move toward a healthier, more active future.

Practical Problem Solving

Functional Neurological Disorder (FND) can present a variety of challenges that affect daily life, including motor or sensory symptoms, cognitive difficulties, emotional distress, and social issues. These challenges can often feel overwhelming, but one way to approach them is through practical problem-solving. Practical problem solving involves breaking down complex issues into manageable parts and applying structured strategies to address them effectively. This approach can empower individuals with FND to regain a sense of control and improve their overall well-being.

In this section, we'll explore how to use practical problem-solving to navigate the difficulties that arise with FND, allowing individuals to create actionable steps that reduce distress and improve functioning.

Why Practical Problem-Solving Matters for FND

Living with FND can involve dealing with both physical symptoms (like tremors, paralysis, or non-epileptic seizures) and psychological challenges (such as anxiety, depression, or frustration). These difficulties can create a cycle where individuals feel stuck, overwhelmed, or unable to take action.

Practical problem-solving helps to:

Break down overwhelming problems into smaller, more manageable pieces.

Increase a sense of control by providing a structured approach to challenges.

Foster a sense of competence and self-efficacy, reinforcing the belief that you can handle difficult situations.

Reduce stress by focusing on solutions rather than on the problem itself.

Improve emotional and physical well-being by taking proactive steps toward resolution.

Steps in Practical Problem-Solving

To effectively solve problems, particularly those related to FND, it's helpful to follow a structured process. The following 5-step approach is a proven method for practical problem-solving:

1. Identify the Problem Clearly

The first step in practical problem-solving is to identify the problem clearly. In the case of FND, the problem could be related to your symptoms, your emotions, your environment, or your interactions with others.

How to Identify the Problem:

Be specific: Try to define the problem as clearly as possible. Instead of saying, "I can't manage my symptoms," say, "I'm finding it difficult to manage my physical symptoms when I try to exercise."

Break it down: Look at the broader issue and break it into smaller, more specific problems. For example, "I feel too tired to go out" could be broken down into: "I'm anxious about being in public with symptoms" and "I lack the energy to leave the house."

Focus on what you can control: FND symptoms may feel uncontrollable at times, but identifying aspects of the situation that you can manage (such as pacing yourself or asking for support) can help you feel empowered.

Example: "I'm struggling with social situations due to my symptoms" can be broken down into:

Feeling embarrassed or self-conscious about the symptoms in public.

Difficulty predicting when symptoms will occur.

Fear of being judged or misunderstood by others.

2. Brainstorm Possible Solutions

Once you've identified the problem, the next step is to brainstorm potential solutions. This stage is about generating as many ideas as possible, without worrying about their feasibility or practicality at first. The goal is to come up with a wide variety of options to tackle the problem.

How to Brainstorm Solutions:

Write down all possible solutions, even if they seem unrealistic at first. The goal is to get creative and not judge your ideas yet.

Consider different perspectives: Think about solutions from different angles—what would your doctor, a friend, or a family member suggest?

Break down larger solutions into smaller steps: For example, instead of thinking "I need to go back to work," brainstorm steps like "Start working from home," or "Speak with my boss about adjusting my workload."

Example: For the problem of feeling too tired to go out:

Take short walks around the block instead of long outings.

Arrange for someone to accompany you for support.

Start by going to quieter places rather than busy ones to reduce sensory overload.

Practice relaxation or breathing exercises before going out to reduce anxiety.

3. Evaluate and Choose the Best Solution

After brainstorming potential solutions, the next step is to evaluate each option. Consider the pros and cons of each one, and weigh the feasibility and effectiveness of the solutions based on your current circumstances, energy levels, and goals.

How to Evaluate Solutions:

Feasibility: Can you realistically implement this solution? Does it fit within your current physical, emotional, and social resources?

Effectiveness: How likely is the solution to resolve the problem? Have you tried it before? What were the results?

Short-term vs. long-term benefits: Does the solution provide a short-term fix or a long-term resolution? Prioritize those that offer lasting benefits or contribute to your overall well-being.

Support: Can you enlist help from others (family, therapists, etc.) to make the solution more manageable?

Example: To address the problem of feeling too tired to go out:

Solution 1: Take short walks (feasible and effective, long-term benefit for physical health).

Solution 2: Ask a family member to accompany you (feasible with support, builds confidence in social situations).

Solution 3: Go to quieter places (can be effective for reducing sensory overload, but may not address underlying anxiety in the long term).

4. Develop a Plan of Action

Once you've selected the best solution, it's time to develop a plan of action. This plan should break down the solution into smaller, achievable steps, with a clear timeline for when you will implement them.

How to Create a Plan of Action:

Set realistic goals: Choose small, achievable steps that you can manage. For example, if you're starting with short walks, begin with 5 minutes per day and gradually increase the time as your stamina improves.

Create a timeline: When will you take the first step? When will you evaluate the success of your solution? Having a timeline helps ensure that you stay on track and assess your progress.

Anticipate obstacles: Consider potential obstacles and plan for them. For example, if you're worried about overexertion, schedule a rest break after the walk.

Example: For addressing fatigue and social withdrawal:

1. Step 1: Start with 5-minute walks at a time of day when you feel most energized (within the next 2 days).

2. Step 2: Invite a family member to join you, so you feel supported and less anxious (within the next week).

3. Step 3: Gradually increase the walk duration as you feel comfortable.

4. Step 4: After 2 weeks, assess how you feel and if you're ready to try visiting a social event with someone for support.

5. Review and Adjust the Plan

The final step in practical problem-solving is to review the outcome of your solution and adjust your plan as needed. It's important to be flexible and open to modifying your approach if things aren't working as expected.

How to Review and Adjust:

Evaluate success: Did the solution help alleviate the problem? If not, what barriers did you encounter?

Make adjustments: If the solution didn't work as planned, try tweaking it or considering a different option from your original brainstorming list.

Celebrate small wins: Even if the solution didn't fully resolve the problem, celebrate any positive steps you've made. Progress is often incremental.

Example: After two weeks of walking and social outings:

Success: You were able to take short walks regularly and felt less anxious about social situations with support.

Adjustment: If the anxiety around being in public is still high, you might consider integrating relaxation techniques or cognitive behavioral therapy (CBT) strategies to manage fears.

Example Scenario: Practical Problem-Solving for FND

Problem: Difficulty managing physical symptoms while trying to return to work.

1. Identify the Problem: I feel anxious about returning to work because I'm worried that my FND symptoms (e.g., tremors or weakness) will make it difficult to complete tasks or be understood by my colleagues.

2. Brainstorm Possible Solutions:

Start working from home to ease back into work.

Ask for flexible work hours to accommodate rest periods.

How to Become More assertive

Living with Functional Neurological Disorder (FND) can present unique challenges, as it often involves fluctuating physical symptoms such as tremors, paralysis, or non-epileptic seizures. It can also impact emotional health, leading to anxiety, frustration, and sometimes feelings of powerlessness. Assertiveness — the ability to express your thoughts, feelings, and needs directly and respectfully — can play a significant role in managing FND and improving your quality of life.

Becoming more assertive is important because it helps you:

Communicate your needs more effectively with healthcare providers, family, friends, and colleagues.

Set boundaries to protect your emotional and physical well-being.

Manage stress by advocating for yourself, reducing the tendency to avoid situations or become passive.

Maintain a sense of control over your life, which can be especially empowering when managing unpredictable symptoms.

In this guide, we will explore how individuals with FND can develop assertiveness to improve their daily lives, relationships, and self-advocacy.

1. Understand Your Rights and Needs

The first step in becoming more assertive, especially when living with FND, is recognizing that you have the right to speak up about your needs and concerns. Your symptoms are real, and you deserve respect, understanding, and accommodations where necessary.

Rights to Recognize:

The right to express your symptoms: Whether you're experiencing physical symptoms (like pain or muscle weakness) or psychological ones (like anxiety or confusion), you have the right to communicate what you're experiencing.

The right to ask for accommodations: If you need adjustments at work, school, or in social situations (like a quiet space or more time for tasks), it's important to assertively request them.

The right to set boundaries: You are not obligated to push yourself beyond your limits or tolerate unhelpful behavior from others. It's okay to say "no" when something feels overwhelming.

Once you understand and accept these rights, you'll be more prepared to speak up for yourself in situations where your needs are not being met.

2. Learn to Recognize and Express Your Symptoms

FND can be challenging because its symptoms can be unpredictable. Sometimes, it's difficult for others to understand what you're going through because they may not be able to see your symptoms or they may fluctuate in severity. Being assertive involves communicating your symptoms clearly, so others understand what you need.

How to Express Your Symptoms Assertively:

Use "I" statements: This helps you take ownership of your experiences while avoiding sounding accusatory. For example:

"I'm feeling very fatigued today, so I need to take a break."

"I experience tremors in my hands, which makes it difficult to hold things."

Be specific and factual: Rather than generalizing, explain exactly what you're feeling or experiencing. For example:

"I'm currently experiencing weakness on my left side, so I need assistance with mobility."

"My vision is blurry, so I might need help reading or navigating."

Provide context when necessary: If you're in a situation where someone might not understand your symptoms (e.g., a new healthcare provider or a friend), briefly explain FND and its impact on your daily life.

By expressing your symptoms clearly, you give others the opportunity to offer support or make accommodations. This proactive communication helps reduce misunderstandings and frustration.

3. Set Clear Boundaries

Living with FND means managing both physical and emotional limits. It's important to establish boundaries that protect your well-being while also being respectful to others. Assertively setting boundaries ensures that you aren't overwhelmed by demands from others that could worsen your symptoms or emotional health.

How to Set Boundaries Assertively:

Recognize your limits: Be aware of when you're reaching your limits — whether it's physical, emotional, or mental. It's okay to take breaks, avoid overexertion, and avoid situations that are too overwhelming.

Communicate your needs: Let others know when you need to step back. For example:

"I need to leave early today because my symptoms are worsening."

"I'm not able to participate in that activity right now because it might trigger my symptoms."

Be firm but polite: When someone asks you to do something you're not able to do, be clear in your response. For instance:

"I'm unable to meet today because of how I'm feeling, but I'd love to reschedule when I'm feeling better."

Use non-verbal communication: Sometimes your symptoms may make it hard to speak, but you can still assert boundaries through gestures or written communication. If someone is asking too much of you, a simple hand gesture or written note can communicate your limits.

By setting and maintaining boundaries, you ensure that you don't push yourself too hard, which can worsen your symptoms or lead to burnout.

4. Practice Saying "No"

Saying "no" can be difficult for anyone, but it's even more challenging when dealing with a chronic condition like FND.

Often, people with FND may feel guilty about saying "no" to others because they worry about disappointing them. However, being able to say "no" assertively is crucial to maintaining your health and well-being.

How to Say "No" Assertively:

Be clear and direct: If you can't do something or don't want to do something, say "no" clearly without apologizing excessively. For example:

"No, I can't make it to the event this week because I need to rest."

"I'm not able to help with that right now, but I appreciate you asking."

Offer an alternative (if possible): If you want to maintain a relationship or help in some way but are unable to fulfill a specific request, offer an alternative. For instance:

"I can't come to the meeting today, but I'm happy to follow up by email tomorrow."

Avoid over-explaining: You don't need to justify why you're saying no. A simple, straightforward response is often enough.

Remember that it's okay to prioritize your health. Saying "no" when you need to is an essential part of self-care, especially when managing FND.

5. Be Honest About Your Limitations

Living with FND may mean that you have limitations in certain areas of your life. Being honest about those limitations with others — whether it's with your employer, family, or friends — is key to maintaining a sense of balance and well-being.

How to Be Honest About Limitations:

Explain your limitations when appropriate: Let others know what you can and cannot do, and be honest about how you're feeling. For example:

"I'm having trouble with walking today, so I need some extra time or assistance."

"I'm feeling overwhelmed by noise and crowds, so I need a quiet space to rest."

Offer solutions: If possible, offer suggestions for how others can support you or work around your limitations. For instance:

"I can't attend the meeting in person, but I can participate by video call."

"I can handle smaller tasks today, but I may need help with larger tasks."

Being honest about your limitations can help others understand your situation better and prevent unnecessary strain on yourself.

6. Communicate with Healthcare Providers Assertively

It's important to be assertive with healthcare providers to ensure you're receiving the right treatment and support for your FND. This can be particularly challenging because FND symptoms are often misunderstood or dismissed by some doctors or specialists. Here's how to advocate for yourself in medical settings:

How to Communicate Assertively with Healthcare Providers:

Prepare for appointments: Before seeing a doctor or therapist, make a list of your symptoms, concerns, and questions. Bring this list with you to the appointment to help guide the conversation.

Be specific about your experiences: Clearly describe your symptoms, how they affect your life, and any changes you've noticed. For example:

"I've noticed increased weakness in my legs, and it's making it hard to walk without assistance."

"I'm feeling very fatigued after short periods of activity, and this is affecting my ability to complete daily tasks."

Ask for clarification: If you don't understand something the doctor is saying, don't hesitate to ask for clarification. It's important that you fully understand your treatment plan.

Request the support you need: Don't be afraid to ask for accommodations, additional referrals, or second opinions if you feel that your needs are not being met.

Assertively communicating with healthcare providers ensures that you are active in your own treatment and that your needs are prioritized.

7. Build Confidence in Self-Advocacy

Asserting yourself may feel uncomfortable at first, especially if you're used to being passive or avoiding conflict. However, practice is key to building confidence in self-advocacy.

Ways to Build Confidence:

Start with small steps: Practice assertiveness in lower-pressure situations before tackling more difficult conversations. For example, start by asserting your needs with friends or family members.

Reflect on successful interactions: After an assertive conversation, take time to reflect on what went well and how you can continue improving. Celebrate your victories, no matter how small.

Seek support: If you find it difficult to be assertive, consider talking to a therapist or counselor who can help you develop and practice these skills.

Role-play scenarios: Practicing assertiveness in role-playing exercises (with a supportive friend or therapist) can help you build confidence and prepare for real-life situations.

Conclusion

Becoming more assertive when living with Functional Neurological Disorder (FND) is a vital skill that can improve your ability to manage symptoms, communicate your needs, and maintain your overall well-being. By understanding your rights, setting boundaries, expressing your needs clearly, and building confidence, you can navigate the challenges of FND in a way that empowers you and enhances your quality of life. Assertiveness helps you regain control over your experiences and ensures that you are treated with respect and understanding by others.

Printed in Great Britain
by Amazon